The Ultimate Cures and Remedies For Acne

The Most Effective, Permanent Solution To Finally Cure Acne For Life

Elizabeth Grace

Table of Contents

Introduction

I want to thank you and congratulate you for purchasing the book, *"The Ultimate Cures and Remedies For Acne: The Most Effective, Permanent Solution To Finally Cure Acne For Life"*.

This book contains proven steps and strategies on how to finally cure your acne or pimple problem and prevent it from coming back.

You no longer have to be embarrassed by your skin problem or forever hide your skin with uncomfortable make-up. This book will also show you how to deal with oily skin which is commonly experienced by acne sufferers. In addition, it will teach you what to do with the scars which inevitably occur after your pimples heal.

Thanks again for purchasing this book, I hope you enjoy it!

Chapter 1 – Acne Basics

Before we discuss how to deal with acne, we must understand how it forms. This is important in order to avoid the frustrations we sometimes experience when we choose an incorrect solution to our problems.

To explain, acne is caused by three factors: excess sebum, excess dead skin cells, and excess bacteria in the skin pores. However, what most people do not know is their acne may have a major cause which is either of the three above. The major cause will determine the kind of acne one suffers from and consequently the best way to deal with it.

Acne can be roughly categorized as mild, moderate or severe. Mild acne is characterized by clogged pores which appear as blackheads and whiteheads. There is very little inflammation in the form of red pimples though these may occasionally sprout up. Moderate acne is characterized by small, inflamed pimples (about the size of an unsharpened pencil point) and it may or may not be accompanied by blackheads and whiteheads. Severe acne is characterized by large and very inflamed pimples which may also be accompanied by the symptoms of mild and moderate acne. Obviously, there are those whose acne may be characterized as in between mild and moderate, and likewise in between moderate and severe, but for our purposes here these characterizations will suffice.

Mild acne is generally caused by excess dead skin cells. The skin is comprised of two layers, the epidermis and dermis. The latter is where capillaries are found which bring nourishment for the skin from the blood. It is also where new skin cells are made. The epidermis is the top layer and is tougher than the dermis since it is built to withstand the sun and wind (though of course only up to a certain degree). As the new skin cells get older, they are pushed up to the epidermis where, once they reach the top layer, they die and flake off. The dust which accumulates in our homes is actually comprised of dead skin cells mixed with other kinds of dirt found in our environment.

The shedding of dead skin cells is a natural process, but as we grow older the skin becomes less efficient in doing this. Instead of being automatically shed, the dead skin cells linger on the surface of the skin where they can mix with the naturally produced sebum or oil produced by our oil glands, or with make-up residues, dirt or other things which are left on the skin due to improper hygiene habits. In time, this mixture will fill up the pores and result in either blackheads or whiteheads. (Blackheads only appear black because the contents of the clogged pore have been exposed to air and have oxidized. The color is not caused by dirt as some people believe.) If you suffer from this kind of acne, then your solution must focus on the reduction of dead skin cells.

Notice that pores can become clogged even without an excess of sebum. That is, people with normal or dry skin can suffer from this type of acne if they do not cleanse their skin properly or regularly remove their dead skin cells. We have to remember that even dry and normal skin produce sebum. Thus, these skin types can still get clogged pores.

Meanwhile, moderate acne is generally caused by excess dead skin cells *and* a small amount of the bacteria Propionibacterium acnes or P acnes for short. The redness one sees in a pimple is actually inflammation. Contrary to what most people believe, inflammation is not a bad thing. It is the body's natural reaction when the white blood cells flood to a certain area to clear up the excessive population of bacteria. The pus which forms and swells up a pimple is comprised of the dead white blood and bacteria cells.

How did P acnes get into the skin pores? It may get there through the hands, a handkerchief, the wind, dust, pillows, and so on. It will be difficult to know how exactly P acnes gets into one's pores, but the fact remains that it does. Once in the pores, it will feed on dead skin cells and sebum and can easily multiply depending on its food supply.

In cases of moderate acne, the sufferer likely has normal or combination skin, i.e. oily only on the forehead, nose and chin, aka the "T-zone". Since the skin does not produce excess sebum, P acnes bacteria have a limited food supply and will not be able to reproduce quickly. This results in less inflamed pimples. However, take note that since P acnes also feeds on dead skin cells, a person with normal or combination skin can find himself suddenly plagued by large pimples if he allows excess dead skin cells to pile up because this will give the bacteria more food and encourage them to multiply.

If you suffer from moderate acne, you need to focus on the reduction of dead skin cells *and* P acnes bacteria. You might also need to reduce the amount of oil produced by your T-zone to further minimize the population of P acnes.

Lastly, severe acne is caused by oily skin, excess dead skin cells and a high population of P acnes. Take note that *all three* must be present or else no pimples or clogged pores will form. It is necessary to clarify this because people often make the mistake of thinking that if they have oily skin, they will inevitably have pimples. Oily skin is not a curse and though there are ways to reduce the skin's oil production, it is possible to live with oily skin but *not* have pimples. We will discuss this further in the succeeding chapters.

Severe acne is generally characterized by large pimples, each of which is about the size of a pencil eraser or possibly even larger. Pimples can become large due to the amount of inflammation caused by an excess of bacteria in one pore, or the inflammation can spread to several pores. The second case can happen when two or three pores which are beside each other become clogged and filled with bacteria. Since these pimples are beside each other, they may appear like one large pimple when in fact they are two or three small ones grouped together. Alternatively, the inflammation might have started in only one pore, but if the amount of bacteria is extremely excessive resulting in an excessive amount of pus, the pore's walls might break resulting in the spread of pus and live bacteria to the other pores.

Severe acne might also be characterized by cystic acne or very large and painful pimples which seem to grow under the skin. This happens when the pores are already clogged but the oil glands continue to produce excessive amounts of oil. If excessive numbers of P acnes also exist, the abundance of food will further swell their already large population. When the body sends white blood cells to counter the growth of P acnes, severe inflammation occurs. Since the population of P acnes is extremely high, the body sends an equally large army of white blood cells. This is why cystic pimples are more inflamed than normal pimples.

You may have *mild* severe acne, in which you only suffer from 5 or so large pimples, or you may have *moderate* severe acne with 10 or so large pimples, or you may have *severe* acne with several large inflamed pimples all over your face. The most severe acne will have mostly cystic pimples. If you suffer mostly from cysts, you have what is more commonly called as "cystic acne".

At this point we must clarify that the occasional large pimple some people get once or twice a year is not severe acne. That may only be a case of their forgetting to wash their face properly or using a product which is not good for their skin. Severe acne is characterized by the regular or consistent development of large pimples. The same may be said about mild and moderate acne. The occasional blackhead, whitehead or small pimple may be due to other factors. That said, obviously you can heal the occasional spot with the same methods described here, but these fortunate people will generally get by with proper hygiene and health habits.

Dealing with severe acne involves using the same methods and medications used for moderate acne, but a higher percentage of the active ingredient is used. It will also help to either temporarily or permanently decrease the skin's sebum production. We will discuss this further in the succeeding chapters.

In this book, we will discuss how you can clear up the three kinds of acne. If you suffer from a "mixed" kind of acne, i.e. both mild in the form of blackheads and whiteheads, and moderate in the form of small pimples, then follow the suggestions given for both kinds of acne.

The *best solution* for your acne is essentially this: *minimize oil, dead skin cells and P acnes bacteria*. The methods and medications will differ depending on the severity of your acne and what works best for your skin.

Chapter 2 – Mild Acne

As we have discussed, mild acne is characterized by blackheads and whiteheads. You may or may not have oily skin as well. If you have oily skin and you need to find ways to control it, check the suggestions listed in chapter 4. In this chapter, since those who suffer from mild acne generally do not have oily skin, we will focus on how to deal with the major symptom of clogged pores.

Since clogged pores are caused by excess dead skin cells mixed with various residues, the solution is to regularly rid the surface of the skin of these substances. Excess dead skin cells can be removed through regular exfoliation while residues can be minimized through proper hygiene. We will discuss each in turn.

Regarding exfoliation, you can choose to do physical exfoliation, chemical or both. Physical exfoliation refers to the use of grainy substances like oatmeal, cornmeal, sugar, plastic beads or even crushed diamonds to scrub away the dead skin cells. You can easily find commercially available facial scrubs in the market today which uses grainy substances to exfoliate or you can make your own facial scrub from ingredients commonly found in your kitchen. Alternatively, you can use your regular facial wash or soap with a facial brush or sponge. If you prefer a professional's touch, you can ask your dermatologist or facialist to give you a microdermabrasion which uses crushed diamond powder and a machine to exfoliate. This last method is generally expensive and must only be done on a monthly basis. Some people find that using facial scrubs at least twice a week gives them the same results as a monthly professional microdermabrasion; however you may prefer the professional treatment if you find it difficult to remember to exfoliate regularly. Ultimately, what you choose will depend on what works for you and your personal preferences.

Chemical exfoliation refers to the use of substances which dissolve dead skin cells which are then washed or wiped away afterwards. Common chemical exfoliants include acids like alpha hydroxy acid, salicylic acid, lactic acid and the various fruit based acids. They also include tretinoin, benzoyl peroxide and various chemicals which can make the skin peel. Commercially available products with chemical exfoliants generally contain only a small percentage of the active ingredient to prevent accidentally burning the skin. If you prefer a deeper exfoliation, you can ask your dermatologist or facialist to give you a chemical peel but this may result in reddened skin which can take up to a week to heal.

Recently, lasers have been used in skin clinics to exfoliate. It is debatable whether lasers count among physical or chemical exfoliants. Most people will say that lasers are chemical exfoliants since the light "burns" the dead skin cells in order to dissolve them.

The third method of exfoliation combines both physical and chemical exfoliation for a more intense effect. For example, you may choose to use a scrub which contains both cornmeal and salicylic acid, or you may use a scrub first then apply a mask, moisturizer or treatment which contains a chemical exfoliant. Your dermatologist or facialist can also give you a microdermabrasion followed by a chemical peel, but take note that this combination might result in more irritation.

If you would like to save money on exfoliants, here are ways to use common ingredients to exfoliate your skin:

- Add cornmeal, oatmeal, or fine sugar to your usual facial wash.

- Make a mask of crushed papaya or strawberries mixed with a little yoghurt. Both the fruit and yoghurt contain acids. Adding yoghurt makes it easier for the crushed fruit to adhere to your skin. Leave the mask on your face for at least 20 minutes.

- Crush two or three aspirins and mix them with a tablespoon of yoghurt. Scrub this on your clean face then leave it for at least 15 minutes. The crushed aspirin is grainy enough to provide physical exfoliation, and it also contains salicylic acid which provides chemical exfoliation.

There are two important things to keep in mind when using exfoliants. First, you must take note of what your skin can and cannot take. It may be normal for the skin to be irritated after the harsher methods of exfoliation which are only done in a professional's clinic, but products which are meant for home use must not give you the same results. If you experience redness or other forms of irritation from an exfoliating product, decrease the frequency of its use. If you use a physical exfoliant which is applied with your fingers, you might need to refrain from applying too much pressure or from scrubbing too long. If you use a chemical exfoliant, you might need to choose one with a lower percentage of the active ingredient.

What you do will depend on what works for you and you can only know this after doing some trial and error testing. If you are not sure how to proceed, you can ask your dermatologist or skin expert. While professionals will also use a trial and error procedure to determine what is best for your skin, they will have the advantage of being able to professionally analyze your skin type in order to weed out products which they know are not applicable for you. For example, they will be able to determine if your skin is sensitive and thus will choose gentle ingredients for you to try.

Second, exfoliation makes the skin more sensitive to the sun, i.e. your skin can easily burn from the sun's rays; hence you must always use a sun protection product even during the days when you do not exfoliate. If this seems like too much trouble, you can remind yourself that regularly using sun protection will help to prevent premature aging and skin cancer.

While regular exfoliation will keep excess dead skin cells at bay, you must also ensure that your skin is regularly cleansed of residues from make-up, dirt and other substances in the environment. Regularly washing your face at least twice a day will suffice if you do not wear make-up. If you wear make-up, you must learn how to remove all traces of it before going to bed. It will also help to use non-comedogenic products or those which have been proven to not clog pores.

Exfoliation and proper cleansing will clean the pores and prevent them from being clogged again. You can expect to find a reduction in clogged pores after two weeks and a major improvement after a month. To prevent your pores from ever being clogged again, you must include these habits in your skin care routine forever. Take note that your skin will never stop producing dead skin cells because that is how it naturally regenerates; thus if you are the sort whose pores regularly get clogged, then exfoliation is how you deal with this tendency. This may be unfortunate, but unless you can change the way your skin works, there is nothing you can do.

Some people complain that if everybody's skin produces dead skin cells, then why do some people never get clogged pores? Perhaps they do but due to regular exfoliation, they prevent this from happening. You can also think of the problem of acne as genetically inherited. Those who have acne-prone skin tend to have relatives who have the same skin type. Indeed, there have been studies which suggest that there is an acne gene. Thus, unless you can find a way to alter your genes, there is nothing you can do. You can either complain about it or simply do something to solve the problem.

If you still think that these habits are too much of a hassle, it may help you to know that they can also prevent premature aging and keep the skin looking radiant.

Chapter 3 – Moderate Acne

In this chapter, we will discuss how to cure and prevent small pimples. If you also suffer from blackheads and whiteheads, you can use the methods described above for mild acne. At any rate, since moderate acne is also caused by excess dead skin cells, you must also exfoliate regularly and maintain proper hygiene habits. People who suffer from moderate acne usually have normal or combination skin, but if you suffer from oily skin, you can check out chapter 4 to know how to deal with this.

There is one difference sufferers of moderate acne must keep in mind when exfoliating. They must not scrub inflamed pimples since this may cause scarring. This can also cause pain when the pimple bursts and the skin is torn off. If you suffer from several pimples scattered all over your face, it is better to use a chemical exfoliant. If you suffer only from a few pimples, then you can use a physical exfoliant but avoid scrubbing on the inflamed pimples.

Together with regular exfoliation and proper cleansing, you must use a product which minimizes the amount of P acnes in the skin pores. The over-the-counter ingredients which you can use against P acnes include benzoyl peroxide, unrefined or virgin coconut oil, and essential oils with anti-bacterial properties like tea tree oil, eucalyptus, lavender, wintergreen and neem. Prescription products include tretinoin and other retinoid formulations, oral antibiotics and the harsher topical anti-bacterial ingredients like azelaic acid and clindamycin. (Note: Countries may differ in what they consider prescription medication. For example, some countries require a prescription for tretinoin while some do not.)

As with exfoliating products, what you use will depend on what works for you and your personal preferences. Benzoyl peroxide and tea tree oil are considered the most effective followed by the other essential oils. Coconut oil is the least effective and is not recommended for oily skin, but it can be used to dilute the various essential oils especially if you have sensitive skin.

These ingredients are available in various forms from cleansers to toners to treatments.

These products will contain the active ingredient in varying strengths. There are also make-up lines made for acne-prone skin which contain anti-bacterial essential oils. You can also use coconut oil and the various essential oils in their pure form.

To use essential oils, apply them pure or diluted with coconut oil directly onto the pimples. Dilute the essential oil if you experience redness or if your eyes and nose find the fumes too irritating. You can also apply the pure or diluted oil all over your face or on pimple prone areas to kill the existing bacteria and prevent pimples from sprouting.

To use coconut oil, choose only unrefined or virgin coconut oil. Refined coconut oil will not have the same anti-bacterial properties. Apply the oil directly on pimples or all over the face as you would a moisturizer. Use at most only 3 drops of oil for your entire face. You should avoid this treatment if you have very oily skin.

Use these products until your pimples clear up. Once your face is clear, you must determine if you need to use anti-bacterial products indefinitely or if can stop using them. (Take note that as explained above, you still need to continue the habit of regular exfoliation and proper cleansing.)

To explain, it is debatable whether you can remove all traces of bacteria in the pores or can just minimize them. There are some people who “outgrow” their pimples and some who suffer from them forever. If you find that you have “outgrown” your pimples and they do not come back even if you never use anti-bacterial products again, then good for you. If you find that your pimples come back after you stop using anti-bacterial products, then you must use them indefinitely.

To check if you have “outgrown” your pimples, start by reducing your use of anti-bacterial products until you only use them twice a week. If you do not get pimples, then you can stop using anti-bacterial products. If you start getting spots again, then you must continue to use them indefinitely. At the very least, use an anti-bacterial facial wash then keep a small amount of anti-bacterial spot treatment for the times when a pimple sprouts.

Chapter 4 – Severe Acne

As discussed in the first chapter, severe acne is cured in the same way as moderate acne. The only difference is a higher percentage of the active ingredient is used since large pimples are caused by a higher population of P acnes in the skin pores. For example, moderate acne sufferers can use 0.25% tretinoin treatment while severe acne sufferers must use 1%.

Unfortunately, using the higher percentage of active ingredient might result in more severe side effects. For example, a higher percentage of tretinoin might result in more peeling and redness. If this is undesirable, you can use the lower percentage but take note that it might take longer for you to see any effects. As I keep saying, what you use will depend on what works for you and your personal preferences.

Those who suffer from severe acne also tend to have very oily skin, i.e. the kind which becomes shiny only 2 hours or less after washing it. If so, then it may help to find ways to minimize or even to temporarily stop oil production. Doing this allows the skin to heal quicker because the P acnes bacteria have less food and thus have less chances of multiplying quickly.

The various ways of dealing with oily skin include the following:

- Oil-free cleansers and other skin products used together with oil blotters throughout the day

- Clay masks to absorb excess oil deep in the pores, or salicylic acid for exfoliation

- Oral contraceptives (only for women)

- Regular use of tretinoin or benzoyl peroxide

- Isotretinoin to temporarily stop oil production

We will discuss each in turn.

Those with naturally oily skin can deal with their skin type by using oil-free cleansers and other skin care products. Cleansers should clean and remove excess oil without drying the skin. It is a mistake to think that oily skin should be cleansed with harsh cleansers. Doing this will only make the skin produce more oil in order to compensate for the dryness.

Oily skin can use anti-aging treatments and sun protection products as long as they are oil-free and non-comedogenic. The best anti-aging treatments for oily skin come in the form of lightweight serums or gels. Sun protection products must provide a matte finish to avoid adding additional shine. Further, make-up products should be specifically made for oily skin. These will have ingredients which soak up oil without clogging the pores.

Since the skin continues to produce oil throughout the day, it would help to have oil blotters to prevent the unattractive shine and also to minimize the food supply for P acnes. It is better to use oil blotters than to apply more make-up to avoid a cakey or mask-like appearance.

Once a week, you can use a clay mask which will absorb the excess oil left in the pores which cannot be reached through normal cleansing. Alternatively, you can use products with salicylic acid. Other exfoliant only exfoliate on the surface of the skin but salicylic acid has been proven to reach down deep into the pores to clear out excess oil.

If you are a woman, you can take oral contraceptives which are proven to make the oil glands produce less oil. Sometimes this alone is enough to clear and prevent moderate acne, but for severe acne it must be used together with other topical medications. Take note that the oil production will go back to normal once you stop taking oral contraceptives. Also, some people might not be able to take this kind of medication due to the side effects.

If you cannot take oral contraceptives and if the use of salicylic acid and oil-free skin care products is not enough, you can try using tretinoin or benzoyl peroxide. Tretinoin can make the skin produce less oil but it might take a long time to see this effect. Benzoyl peroxide has the triple advantage of minimizing P acnes, exfoliating and minimizing oil production. This is why it is the most recommended anti-acne medication. As with oral contraceptives, oil production will return to normal once the medication is stopped.

If all these methods still do not work for you, the last resort is isotretinoin which is more commonly known as the brand name Accutane. What this medication does is to completely shut down the oil glands to allow the most severe acne to heal. Unfortunately, once the medication is stopped, the oil glands will return to normal and acne might begin again.

If severe acne might return after using isotretinoin, then why use it at all? It must be clarified that isotretinoin is only used for the most severe cases characterized by extremely large pimples, especially cystic acne, all over the face and possibly even the neck. Recall that cystic acne occurs because of excessive amounts of sebum and excessive amounts of P acnes. If you can completely stop the production of sebum, you can stop the overproduction of P acnes. Once the isotretinoin medication is completed, the population of P acnes will (hopefully) also be brought down to a manageable population. After isotretinoin, acne can be prevented through the continued use of regular strength acne medications.

You cannot use isotretinoin forever since it has severe side effects. Only the other methods of oil control can be used indefinitely although salicylic acid and tretinoin must be stopped during pregnancy. If those with very oily skin think that they will have to battle excess sebum and acne forever, it may help to remind them that the skin becomes 10% dryer every decade. It might also help them to know that oily skin by itself does not cause acne. For acne to form, excess dead skin cells and P acnes must also be present. Since these two can be managed, it follows that acne can also be managed.

Chapter 5 – Acne Aftermath

Whether you are constantly battling acne or you seem to have "outgrown" it, you still need to deal with the aftermath in the form of acne scars. There are two kinds of acne scars: permanent and temporary. Let us discuss each in turn.

The first kind of acne scarring includes the embedded and icepick scars, and other varieties which are characterized by a permanent indentation on the skin's surface. These usually occur due to large or cystic pimples which cause permanent damage in the dermis. These are considered permanent scars because they will not go away on their own. This does not mean, however, that they cannot be removed through dermatological procedures.

The easiest way to deal with permanent scars is to simply minimize their appearance by making them less deep. This is done through regular exfoliation. The edges of the scar can become less defined as well after several months of exfoliation.

For more dramatic results, you can opt to have dermatological procedures like lasers which provide a deeper exfoliation and also encourage the dermis to repair itself. Through these procedures the skin can return to its normal unmarred state. Take note, however, that it can become scarred again if measures are not taken to prevent the acne from coming back.

If you want a temporary solution, you can fill up the embedded part with thick concealer then cover the whole scar with foundation. This is a timely process which requires a lot of skill to avoid making the concealer look obvious, but if you have a special occasion where looking your best is important, it may be worthwhile to have your acne scars camouflaged. Otherwise, this method is too time-consuming.

Most people find that it is best to simply learn to live with their permanent acne scars. If you are not bothered by them or if your self-esteem is not affected, then this might be the best solution for you. If you are extremely bothered by them, it is best to consult with your dermatologist since she will be able to give you the best solution to your problem. If you decide to do this, be prepared to shell out a lot of money especially if you have extensive scarring. If you are not able to afford expensive procedures, then at the very least continue to exfoliate regularly to make your scars look less obvious.

The second kind of acne scarring includes dark brown or red spots. This is a normal occurrence after the skin has been damaged. These are temporary scars because they will eventually fade even if left alone. However, most people would prefer to hasten their fading.

The best way to do this is through exfoliation. Since you regularly remove the top cells on the surface of the epidermis, you will also remove the discolored cells which form the dark spots.

Another way to hasten the removal of spots is through bleaching them. You can use any of the brightening or whitening products available in the market. The best products will have vitamin C and/or niacinamide as their active ingredient. However, make sure that these products do not cause acne or else you will only make your problem worse.

Since vitamin C can cause acne scars to fade, you can opt to use lemon (or other strong citrus fruit) juice directly on the spots. Use the juice like you would a toner, or else you can rub a slice of the fresh fruit over the spots.

Conclusion

Thank you again for purchasing this book!

I hope this book was able to help you to cure and prevent your acne.

The next step is to try out the suggestions listed here to see what works for you.

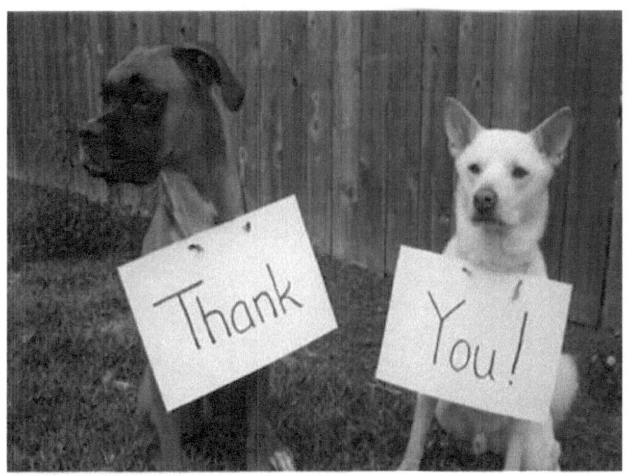

Finally, if you enjoyed this book, then I'd like to ask you for a favor, would you be kind enough to leave a review for this book on Amazon? It'd be greatly appreciated!

Thank you and good luck!

www.ingramcontent.com/pod-product-compliance
Lightning Source LLC
Chambersburg PA
CBHW051405250726
48656CB00006B/2277

* 9 7 8 1 9 7 3 1 6 4 4 6 3 *